Sinus Survival
A Complete Guide To Caring For America's Most Common Ailment

Dr. Robert S. Ivker

Illustrations by
Eileen Rudnick

A publication of Whole Health Press

Revised edition © 1989

First printing November 1988
Second printing February 1989

ISBN: 0-9621845-0-0

Cover photograph: A typical winter day in Denver, Colorado. Air quality on this day was rated "acceptable." Photo by Robert S. Ivker

Acknowledgments

Thanks to the many patients who taught me about sinuses.

Dedication

To my father, Morris, whose love of medicine started me on my present path.

Table of Contents

Introduction.................................5

1. What Are Sinuses?..........................7

2. What Makes Sinuses Sick?...................12

   The Common Cold.......................12
   Cigarettes.............................13
   Air Pollution..........................15
   Dry Air................................18
   Cold Air...............................19
   Allergy................................19
   Occupational Hazards...................20
   Dental Problems........................20
   Emotional Stress.......................21

3. Recognizing a Sick Sinus: Acute and Chronic 22

   Acute Sinusitis........................22
      Head Congestion....................23
      Yellow Mucus.......................23
      Extreme Fatigue 25
      Headache and Facial Pain 26
      Fever..............................28
      Nasal Congestion and Rhinitis......28
      Sore Throat........................28
      Laryngitis.........................29
      Cough..............................29
   Chronic Sinusitis......................31

4. Treating Acute Sinusitis 34

    Traditional Medical Methods 34
    Antibiotics 35
    Decongestants 37
    Analgesics (Pain Relievers) 40
    Moisture 41
    Cough Suppressants 44
    Hydration and Bed Rest 44
    Holistic Methods 45

5. When Sinusitis Coexists with Other
    Medical Conditions 53

    The Common Cold 53
    Acute Otitis Media (Middle Ear Infection) 53
    Allergic Rhinitis (Nasal Allergy) 55
    Bronchitis and Pneumonia 56
    Asthma 57

6. Treating Chronic Sinusitis 59

    Air Cleaners 60
    Decongestants 61
    Moisture 61
    Peppermint Oil 62
    Vitamins 63
    Diet 64
    Exercise 64
    Nasalcrom and Cortisone Sprays 65
    Surgery 67
    Conclusion 69

Introduction

"**Sinus survival**" — it sounds rather ominous. Is the problem actually that serious? After fifteen years as a family physician on the "front lines" of medicine, and having spent the past ten of those years with a sinus condition myself, I am convinced we are dealing with a rapidly growing worldwide epidemic. In the course of this text, I will offer my explanation for this phenomenon and for why it is becoming such a challenge to maintain healthy sinuses.

In the summer of 1981, the National Center for Health Statistics published its latest findings. Surprisingly, for the first time in the center's statistic-taking history, chronic sinusitis was now the number one chronic disease in the United States. It had become more common than arthritis. Why? That they did not explain. In their most recent findings (1983-85), it is still the most prevalent disease, affecting 31.2 million Americans, nearly one of every eight people in this country..

Since that statistic was published, my own practice, on the outskirts of Denver, Colorado, has reflected this burgeoning problem. During the past five years, acute sinusitis has consistently been the most common diagnosis that we have seen in our office. What I've learned from being responsible for the care of more than 20,000 of these patients is that this condition is not easily recognized by either doctor or patient, and that conventional methods of treating sinuses are becoming increasingly less effective. So, that friend of yours who's been complaining of "this terrible cold" that he's had for the past three weeks may in fact not have a cold at all, but probably has acute sinusitis.

The primary purpose of this book is to help people

care for their own sinuses. I have always believed that an important part of Family Practice is patient education. There is no doubt that this book will do a much more thorough job of educating than I could do during a short office visit. Therefore, anyone who reads the book and follows its suggestions should be quite capable of diagnosing and treating (with the possible exception of prescription drugs) his own sinusitis, both acute and chronic.

The book is written for medical professionals and nonmedical people alike. It is based almost entirely upon medical science. During the past few years, I have become familiar with several holistic methods for treating acute sinusitis, which I will also present. Medicine today considers chronic sinusitis to be incurable. I have attempted to provide a fresh perspective and innovative methods for dealing with this problem, which is affecting the quality of life of millions of people all over the world.

Chapter 1

What Are Sinuses?

The sinuses are air-filled cavities located behind and around the nose and eyes. They are medically referred to as the paranasal sinuses. There are usually four pairs — one set for each side of the head. The pairs may be asymmetrical in size and shape.

The sinuses are identified as frontal, maxillary, sphenoid, and ethmoid (Figure A). The frontal sinuses lie above the eyes just above the nose and behind the forehead. The maxillaries, the largest of the sinuses, are pyramid-shaped cavities located behind each cheekbone. The ethmoids are multicompartmental sinuses behind the maxillaries and between the bony orbits of the eyes. They are complex labyrinths of small air pockets. The sphenoids are situated deep in the skull behind the nose, slightly below the ethmoids. The ethmoidal, sphenoidal, and maxillary sinuses are all present at birth, although the latter do not reach full development until sixteen to twenty-one years of age. The frontal sinuses are not present until the age of eight.

Each sinus is connected to the nasal passage by a thin duct about the size of a pencil lead (Figure B). The ducts of the maxillaries are located at the top of the sinus, making drainage difficult and blockage easy. A series of small ducts in the nasal wall drain the ethmoid sinuses, and these openings are easily blocked. The openings of the ducts are called ostia.

The same tissue, called respiratory epithelium, lines all of the sinuses, the nose, and the lungs. In fact, these three are all part of the respiratory tract (Figure C), that system of the body involved with the essential function

8

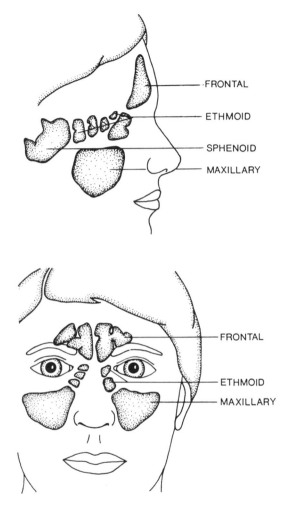

LOCATION OF SINUSES

FIGURE A

of breathing. The outermost part of the epithelium is called the mucosa, which is a mucous membrane. On the surface of this membrane are cilia (microscopic hairlike filaments) that are in constant sweeping motion.

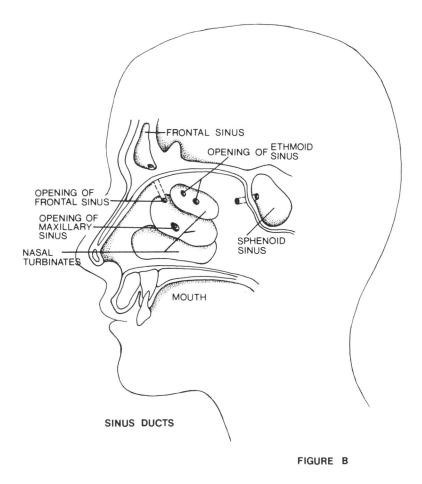

FRONTAL SINUS

OPENING OF ETHMOID SINUS

OPENING OF FRONTAL SINUS

OPENING OF MAXILLARY SINUS

NASAL TURBINATES

SPHENOID SINUS

MOUTH

SINUS DUCTS

FIGURE B

The mucous membrane and its cilia provide a good defensive mechanism against infections. The entire mucus (watery discharge) covering of the maxillary sinus is normally cleared every ten minutes. The membrane produces between a pint and a quart of mucus daily. The mucus traps particles entering the nasal passage for the cilia to sweep toward the back of the nose, where the particles are swallowed and destroyed by stomach acids.

No one within the medical community seems able to scientifically state the exact function of the sinuses.

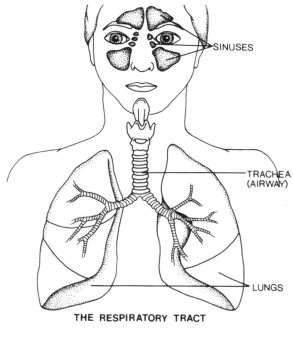

SINUSES

TRACHEA
(AIRWAY)

LUNGS

THE RESPIRATORY TRACT

FIGURE C

(There is agreement, however, that they lighten the weight of the skull). By virtue of their location and structure (anatomy) and the microanatomy and function of the mucous membrane, most physicians would agree with the following conclusions. All these conclusions have frequently been alluded to in the medical literature, although never proven in a laboratory.

The sinuses, along with the nose, as the upper part of the respiratory tract, *serve as the body's chief protector of the lungs.* They do this by acting as a *"filter"* — helping to defend against viruses, dirt and dust particles, allergens, and anything else in the air that would be of no benefit to the lungs; as a *"humidifier"* — by moistening dry air that would be irritating to the lungs; and as a *"temperature regulator"* — by cooling excessively hot air and warming extremely cold air that would be a shock to the lungs. Our lungs are the primary vehicle through which our bodies obtain oxygen — the most vital element in maintaining good health and life itself.

The sinuses, as the body's leading defenders against injury and/or illness to the lungs, have been neglected both by the medical community and by its patients. Think about a quarterback on the football field whose offensive line is weak and beginning to break down. He may not be killed, literally, but what about his health and the quality of his life? Our sinuses are being assaulted and are beginning to deteriorate. The health of our lungs, and ultimately our bodies, is at stake. Let us see how we might help preserve good health by reinforcing our first line of defense, the sinuses.

Chapter 2

What Makes Sinuses Sick?

The factors that will be discussed in this chapter have the potential to adversely affect any sinus, but the weakened sinus and the person who has had previous sinus problems are most susceptible to these things: the common cold, cigarettes, air pollution, dry air, cold air, fumes, allergies, and emotional stress.

The Common Cold

The story of what often becomes a lifetime of "sinus problems" usually begins with the common cold. Normally, air and mucus flow freely along the ducts connecting the nose and sinuses. Trouble starts when the system becomes obstructed, usually by a cold. This obstruction occurs as a result of inflammation and swelling of the nasal mucous membrane. The cold virus inactivates the cilia of the nasal membrane, causing the mucus in the nose to stagnate rather than flow (Figure D). As a result, the mucus being produced in the sinuses cannot drain properly, and the sinuses become a breeding ground for bacteria. This pooling of stagnant mucus can easily result in a sinus infection, especially in individuals who have had such infections previously.

Through the early and mid-1970s, I treated many patients who had nothing more than a "bad cold." However, by the late seventies and especially early eighties, patients with the common cold became less frequent visitors to my office. They were being replaced by patients who greeted me with complaints like, "Doctor, I have had this cold for the past two weeks now" (or three weeks or several months, or in a few cases, a year or more!). These people usually had sinusitis, and not until they had completed at least a ten-day course of antibiotics were they able to rid themselves of their "cold." It also became quite apparent that subsequent to their first infection, those who had never before had a sinus infection were now frequently returning with the same problem. As a result of that first bout with sinusitis, the mucous membrane and especially the cilia are left in a somewhat damaged and weakened state. For many, the membrane never completely recovers, especially in an environment that is harsh on the sinuses. What I have been observing with increasing frequency is that one "bad cold" can ultimately result in a permanently weak sinus, i.e., chronic sinusitis. This impaired sinus then becomes much more susceptible to additional infections, as a result of a cold or any of the other risk factors that I will now describe.

Cigarettes

Whenever a patient with a sinus infection returns to my office two or more weeks after completing a course of antibiotics and complains to me, "Doctor, I'm not any better," my first response is always the question, "Have you been smoking?" Invariably, the patient answers yes. It is extremely difficult to have healthy sinuses if you smoke cigarettes. Nicotine paralyzes the cilia. I would be hard pressed to name anything more harmful to the body's air filter than smoke of any kind that is inhaled or exhaled through the nose. Cigarette smoke is most often involved, but cigar, pipe, campfire, and cooking smoke are also frequent villains. Remember, too, that marijuana and especially cocaine are quite harmful to the nasal mucous membrane.

If you are curious what smoke does to the sinuses, take a look at a used cigarette filter. It will give you some idea of what is happening not only to the sinuses, but to the lungs as well. What is occurring at the tissue level is that the smoke causes irritation of the mucous membrane. The weaker the sinus (i.e., usually one that has been infected previously), the greater the level of irritation. The greater the irritation, the more inflamed the mucous membrane becomes. Inflammation of the mucous membrane results in its swelling, increased mucus secretion, and damage to the cilia. This swelling can potentially cause obstruction of the sinuses, which then produces a condition in the sinuses very similar to that created by the common cold (Figure D).

The principle described here of body fluids being obstructed holds true for almost any part of the human body. Whether it is the bladder, bowel, lung, kidney, or middle ear space, when fluids or secretions are unable to drain normally, the potential for infection is high. This likely scenario of infection in the sinuses can be triggered not only by the common cold and cigarette smoke, but almost all of the other factors that I will mention later in this chapter. This is a theory that the medical establishment has not yet proven. It is presently beyond the scope of science to microscopically observe what is happening to the mucous membrane in someone's sinus as it is being suffocated with smoke. However, as with the speculation on the function of the sinuses, this theory, too, would have strong support among most physicians.

For those of you who are sinus sufferers and do not smoke, and therefore may not have been paying close attention, I am sorry to say that even you are not immune to the problems generated by smoke. Studies in recent years have shown that nonsmokers who live or work with smokers are adversely affected. New laws

15

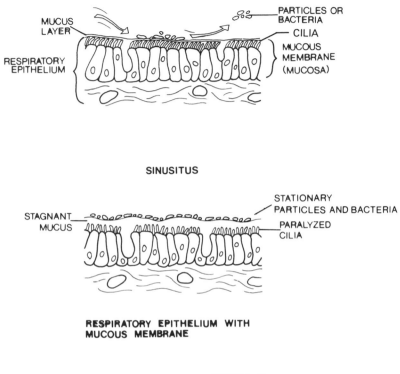

HEALTHY

MUCUS LAYER — PARTICLES OR BACTERIA — CILIA — MUCOUS MEMBRANE (MUCOSA) — RESPIRATORY EPITHELIUM

SINUSITUS

STAGNANT MUCUS — STATIONARY PARTICLES AND BACTERIA — PARALYZED CILIA

RESPIRATORY EPITHELIUM WITH MUCOUS MEMBRANE

FIGURE D

that prohibit cigarette smoking in public places are helping, but we have a long way to go in this endeavor.

Air Pollution

I was struck by a comment made by one of the Apollo astronauts several years ago following his mission. He said that the most disturbing part of his flight was seeing a grayish haze over almost every land mass on the Earth. What was this mysterious ugly blanket covering our beautiful planet? No explanation was given. One could only guess at the answer.

However, living in Denver gave me a good clue. The

"Mile-High City," one of this country's most polluted metropolitan areas, is often covered by a thick brownish-gray pall of smog known locally as "the brown cloud." Most cities in the world are similarly afflicted with significant air pollution. In mountainous areas where temperature inversions are frequent; in cities where diesel fuel is used extensively, especially in Europe; in the heavily industrialized northeast corridor of the United States, the problem of air pollution is even more acute. Almost every country in the world is now familiar with this rapidly growing dilemma. Is it possible that it has reached such immense proportions that it is visible from space? Even more important, what is this filthy air doing to the human beings who have created the problem?

Since the early 1970s, the incidence of acute sinusitis has risen dramatically in Denver. In my practice, it has consistently been the most common ailment since 1981. Is it only a coincidence that air pollution has undergone a similar meteoric rise during the same period of time? The pollution is most acute from mid-November to mid-January, when temperature inversions (warm air aloft trapping cold air and pollutants near the ground) are most common. This also happens to be the time of year when we see the greatest number of sinus infections. Many people who work in center city or in other high pollution areas are aware of the connection between their sinus congestion and sinus headaches on particularly bad pollution days.

There is convincing data to implicate carbon monoxide as the most dangerous element of air pollution. Why? Because in high enough concentrations, it is capable of killing people with weak hearts and lungs. It is also the most often measured component of air pollution. But carbon monoxide is an odorless and colorless gas. What is that stuff that we can see — the brown cloud — and what is it doing to the sinuses of us healthy people when we breathe it?

Visible pollution consists primarily of the following elements: particulates, oxides of sulfur, oxides of nitrogen, ozone, and hydrocarbons. Particulates are tiny particles of solid material — dust, sand, cinders, ashes — found in the atmosphere. They come from a variety of sources, including roads, farm fields, construction sites, power plants, fireplaces, wood-burning stoves, diesel and car exhaust. When inhaled, larger particles are known to lodge in the nose and sinuses. After all, what is a filter for? Oxides of sulfur, especially sulfur dioxide (a colorless gas with a pungent odor), are typically found in combination with particulates. They are emitted mainly by coal- and oil-fired power plants, refineries, and industry. Sulfur oxides are also the responsibility of the filtering sinuses and are easily absorbed across their mucosal lining. Unfortunately, in protecting the lungs from this toxic substance, there is a price to be paid. Studies have shown that sulfur oxides have an intensely irritating effect on the bronchial mucosa (same type of tissue as in sinuses), resulting in damage to the cilia and initiation of bronchitis. So if sulfur oxides can cause bronchitis in the lungs, is it too great an assumption to postulate that they can also cause sinusitis?

Nitrogen oxides, particularly nitrogen dioxide, are the principal constituents of photochemical smog (a reddish-brown gas). They are emitted by combustion. Sources include home heating, wood burning, power plants, automobiles, and aircraft. Like sulfur oxides, nitrogen oxides cause bronchial irritation and ciliary paralysis. They are also capable of impairing the immune defenses against bacterial and viral infection. Nitrogen dioxide can also form nitrates, which are particulates.

Ozone results from chemical reactions in the air involving certain pollutants. Hydrocarbons from car exhaust, stored gasoline, solvents, cleaning fluids, and ink react in sunlight with nitrogen oxides in the atmosphere to form ozone. Although present in smaller concentrations than nitrogen oxides, ozone is much more potent in producing similar toxic effects.

Hydrocarbons are evaporated or incompletely burned organic compounds. The largest sources of hydrocarbons in the atmosphere include internal combustion engines, certain industrial processes (such as coke ovens in steel mills), and evaporation of liquids (such as gasoline in fuel transfers, and industrial and household solvents). Hydrocarbons are known to be highly irritating to mucous membranes.

In fact, every component of air pollution has already been scientifically shown to be harmful to the lungs. But conspicuous by its absence in the medical and scientific literature is mention of the chief protector of the lungs — the sinuses. There is mounting evidence that the air that most of us on this planet are breathing is unhealthy. Although in most cases this will not prove to be a fatal problem, it has already begun to have an insidious effect upon the quality of life of most urban dwellers. It is my firm conviction that as urban sprawl and development continue to exacerbate the global problem of air pollution, it will become an ever-increasing challenge to maintain healthy sinuses.

Dry Air

An important function of the sinuses is to humidify the air we breathe; a person with weak sinuses may therefore have a problem in situations with an abundance of dry air. Moist air is very helpful for the proper functioning of the mucous membrane. Although usually synonymous with hot air, dry air occurs in conjunction with other phenomena as well. Dry air is associated with

— arid or semiarid climate
— forced hot air heating systems; they not only dry, but give the sinuses more filtering to do
— air conditioning, especially in cars
— wind
— mountains: the higher the elevation, the drier the air
— wood-burning stoves, the most drying of all

Cold Air

Although the moisture content of cold air is generally much higher than dry air, the shock of cold temperatures to the mucous membrane of an impaired sinus can cause significant irritation and ciliary injury.

Allergy

People who have nasal allergies (hay fever) and asthma are very susceptible to sinus infections. The same basic process takes place as I have previously described with the common cold and cigarette smoke. The nasal and sinus mucosa are extremely sensitive, i.e., hypersecretory. When an allergic reaction takes place there is swelling of the mucosa and obstruction of the sinuses.

Many people claim they are "allergic" to cigarette smoke, or dust, or some other irritant in the air. Most of the time they are not really describing an allergy, but an extreme sensitivity of the mucous membrane. This sensitivity causes a similar end result in the nose, stuffiness and mucus drainage, but the process is a bit different. Actual nasal allergies are usually caused by airborne pollen from grass, trees, weeds, flowers, molds, and animal dander (cats, dogs, horses, etc.). In many areas of the United States, these allergies are the major contributors to sinus problems. However, be aware that often the individual complaining of a "year-round allergy problem" actually has chronic sinusitis.

Occupational Hazards

A job that involves any of the aforementioned factors — any type of dirty, dry, extremely hot, or extremely cold air — would be considered a high risk to the sinuses. In my experience, those at highest risk include

- auto mechanics
- construction workers — especially carpenters, who are also the highest risk group for ethmoid sinus cancer in the United States
- painters
- airport and airline personnel — mechanics, maintenance workers, baggage handlers, flight attendants, and even pilots
- white-collar workers in offices where there are one or more smokers
- policemen
- firemen
- parking garage attendants
- professional cyclists*

Dental Problems

After birth, the roots of the teeth and the maxillary sinus come into close proximity; at times they are separated only by paper-thin bone or sinus mucosa. Because of this proximity, periapical abscesses or periodontitis of the upper teeth may extend into the sinus cavity and cause maxillary sinusitis. Minor trauma or injury, dental instrumentation, extraction, or displacement of a chronically inflamed tooth can lead to perforation of the sinus cavity.

The incidence of dental-related sinusitis in children is unknown but probably significant, particularly in ado-

---

* When I worked as the team physician for the 7-Eleven cycling team during the 1986 Coors International Bicycle Classic, a total of five riders in the competition, including Eric Heiden of 7-Eleven, had to drop out due to sinus infections — this in spite of the fact that professional cyclists are the most physically fit human beings I have ever known.

lescents. In adults, possibly 10 percent of maxillary sinus infections are thought to be of dental origin.

Emotional Stress

Emotional stress is probably the single most important determinant in whether someone develops a sinus infection. All the other factors I have described in this chapter have the *potential* for adversely affecting the sinuses. But what is it that triggers that potential? Why is it that a person with weak sinuses can be exposed to the same "risky" conditions many times but only occasionally develops a sinus infection? I am convinced that stress is usually the answer.

In the past couple of years, science has demonstrated in several studies that emotional stress does indeed have an important influence on the body's immune system. This research has even implicated stress as one of the possible causes of cancer. Peace of mind, the mind/body connection, and the vital role played by both emotional and spiritual well-being are becoming a focus in the "enlightened medicine" of the future.

Chapter 3

Recognizing a Sick Sinus: Acute and Chronic

Throughout this book I use the term "sinusitis" to refer to sinus problems in general. This word encompasses two distinctly different medical diagnoses: acute sinusitis and chronic sinusitis.

ACUTE SINUSITIS

Acute sinusitis is another way of saying "sinus infection." This is the problem that usually requires medical attention. I've already mentioned that the common cold is most often the cause of a sinus infection, so let's look at this a bit more closely.

Usually the person who's had negligible previous sinus problems will notice that his cold just won't quit after about seven to ten days; or that the symptoms of the cold have actually gotten much worse; or that the cold was almost gone for one to two weeks and now it's back again. After close questioning it's apparent that the "cold" never really went away.

In people with already weak sinuses (caused by previous sinus infections), the common cold usually results in problems occurring much sooner. They might notice the typical symptoms of a sinus infection arising in only two to three days. The underlying condition of the sinuses will usually determine how soon the symptoms appear. The important thing to keep in mind is that a common cold very often precedes the onset of acute sinusitis. Its presence somewhere in the story of one's illness will help in the recognition of a sick sinus.

What else are we looking for? Are these symptoms different for adults than for children (under the age of twelve)? The answer to the latter question is yes. The most common symptoms are as follows, with the first three being present in almost every adult case of a sinus infection.

Head Congestion

Most people describe this symptom as "fullness" or "a stuffy head." Their nose may or may not be stuffy as well. This symptom is most obvious in the morning upon arising from bed. It is often relieved, although not eliminated, by a hot shower. One may also notice that voice, smell, and taste are somewhat altered. These symptoms, however, are more subtle than the primary one of head congestion. There is a very definite awareness of a fullness in the head or a dull ache behind or above the eyes. If present, it's quite obvious.

Yellow Mucus

This is the question that seems to make patients most uncomfortable: "What color is your mucus?" The usual response, accompanied by a grimace, is, "Eww, I never look at it!" I ask this question for two locations — the nose, and more importantly, the back of the throat. The classic presentation of acute sinusitis, which one usually does not see in an adult, is yellow (actually a yellow/green) mucus coming from one nostril. Children with a sinus infection usually have this colored mucus running from their nose. However, if it's not (no pun intended), it can sometimes make the diagnosis difficult, since most kids are not great nose-blowers. Sniffing actually makes matters worse, since it tends to suck bacteria into the sinus. I usually try to have them blow their nose in the exam room, while I'm there. If you are checking your child at home, please remember to use white tissues; yellow won't help at all. Sinusitis is so often missed in children that in a recent article in a pediatric journal, it was stated that almost 25 percent of all diagnosed upper respiratory tract infections (the common cold) in kids were actually cases of acute sinusitis.

In adults, if it's yellow from the nose, that will help in making the diagnosis. But in many cases it is either clear or white mucus, or there is no mucus at all from the nose. It seems that in most cases of acute sinusitis, the infected or yellow mucus drains down the back of the throat. People are most aware of this in the morning, when they get out of bed and spit into the sink some of the mucus they've collected during the night. This first morning mucus specimen is helpful in making the diagnosis, but it can be present without acute sinusitis. Therefore, the most important question I ask an adult is, "Are you spitting out yellow mucus during the rest of the day, other than first thing in the morning?" Unfortunately, most people will respond with "I swallow it," or "It's not convenient to spit it out," or the old standby, "I never look at it!" If I'm still suspicious of a sinus infection, then I'll ask if they're even aware of mucus dripping down the back of the throat. If they're not aware of this occurring during the day, then I'll go back to "How about when you wake up in the morning?" Often I'll see patients who aren't aware of mucus drainage, but when I look at their throat, there is a thick yellow band of mucus coming down from their sinuses.

I've spent a lot of time on this topic not because I enjoy discussing "gross" subjects, as my daughter Julie would say, but because it is extremely helpful in making the diagnosis. There are very few objective physical signs of acute sinusitis, and this one is consistently present. Many ENT (ear, nose, and throat) specialists might find yellow mucus to be a bit too indefinite. They like to confirm their diagnosis with a sinus X-ray. However, the X-ray costs almost $40 (more than the usual office visit to a family doctor or pediatrician) and it is extremely inconsistent (often people will have every symptom of a sinus infection and the X-ray will be normal); thus it is impractical at best.

Extreme Fatigue

There is hardly a sick patient I can think of who doesn't complain of some degree of fatigue. Most people, even if they're not ill, would admit to being tired for some part of the day. Therefore, I'd like to emphasize the word "extreme," and note that I'm talking about a definite change in normal energy level.

In addition to inquiring about the nasal and head symptoms that are usually mentioned by the patient, I always ask the question, "Does your whole body feel sick in some way?" or "Do you feel especially tired?" The answer is frequently yes. This fatigue illustrates the point that acute sinusitis is a systemic illness, i.e., one that affects the entire being. These people are sick all over. The medical term that best describes this phenomenon is "malaise," meaning a feeling of general discomfort. It's often accompanied by significant irritability. But in addition to this feeling, people with sinus infections usually are sleeping more at night, having some difficulty getting through a full day at work, or perhaps even taking unaccustomed naps. In people who exercise regularly, the change in energy level will be even more evident.

At times, fatigue may even be patients' chief complaint. The bad cold that they had was as long as two or three months ago, and "I just haven't been myself since." These people do not come in complaining of the cold that they still have. Most of the time they think they're finished with it. But in fact, if asked, they'll admit to a stuffy head in the morning and occasional yellow mucus that they have to spit out. These patients pose a tough diagnostic challenge to the physician, as some of them have been tired for so long they have no recollection of any physical illness. I have seen them frequently misdiagnosed with anything from depression to menopause. A few days of antibiotics, however, can do what months of estrogen were unable to do.

The picture presented by acute sinusitis can vary greatly — some people are very sick, others minimally uncomfortable. But you can usually depend on these four elements to make a definitive diagnosis in an *adult:* a preceding cold, head congestion, postnasal yellow mucus, and extreme fatigue. In a *child* the most common symptoms are nasal yellow mucus, fever, foul-smelling breath, and cough.

The following symptoms are not quite as consistent as these first four, but are frequently present.

Headache and Facial Pain

I've combined these two because it's often difficult to differentiate between them. With acute sinusitis, pain and sometimes swelling will occur in the region of the affected sinus (Figure E). For instance, an infected maxillary sinus will cause pain in the cheek (sometimes swelling too), under the eye, and/or in the teeth of the upper jaw, particularly the molars. At times, the tooth pain may be so severe as to prompt a visit to the dentist.

Infected ethmoid sinuses produce pain between and behind the eyes; frontals, in the forehead and over the eyes; and sphenoids, a generalized pain, deep in the head, which becomes aggravated whenever your head is

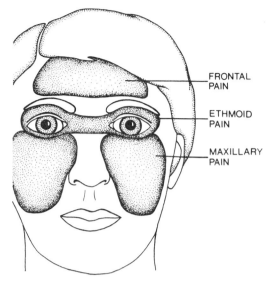

LOCATION OF SINUS PAIN IN ACUTE SINUSITIS

FIGURE E

jarred (as when your heel strikes hard against the ground in walking). Sphenoid pain can often be present as a headache in the back of the head at the base of the skull.

Children may have facial pain accompanied by swelling of the orbit of the eye that involves the upper eyelid, lower lid, or both. Gradual in onset, the swelling is most obvious in the early morning shortly after arising. The swelling may decrease or even disappear during the day, only to reappear the following day.

I should note that some of the most incapacitating headaches I've encountered have resulted from infected frontal sinuses. Sinus headaches tend to worsen when you bend your head forward or lie down. Hence, they often feel worse in the morning after you've lain in bed for hours, and ease somewhat later in the day.

Fever

This is much more common in children than adults. When it's present in an adult, it's usually low-grade (less than 101° F). However, it's not uncommon to see kids run high fevers (103° to 105° F) with acute sinusitis. Often it's early in the course of the infection, and other symptoms are not yet obvious, making the diagnosis difficult. The point here is that because fever accompanies so many different infections, it can't be considered an important diagnostic symptom. However, if I'm suspicious of sinusitis, fever can be a helpful sign in confirming the diagnosis along with the other symptoms that are present.

Nasal Congestion and Rhinitis

This simply means a stuffy and runny nose. We already know that these are the primary symptoms of the common cold and that a cold usually precedes acute sinusitis. Therefore, it's quite common to have an overlapping of the two infections. The important things to keep in mind are that, in adults, stuffiness is more prominent with sinusitis than the runny nose, and it is often present on only one side of the nose. With children the yellow nasal discharge can be copious. Also, with a cold, draining mucus is usually clear and/or white and thin and/or watery, while with sinusitis it's thick and yellow.

Sore Throat

This is probably the most common complaint in any family doctor's office. There are a variety of causes, but a substantial number of sore throats result from postnasal mucus drainage down the back of the throat and mouth breathing. When this occurs, it does not always mean the underlying problem is sinusitis, but there are a few key points to investigate to find out if it is. A sore throat from sinusitis is usually not consistent throughout the day — it is much worse in the morning upon awakening. In fact, the sore throat itself can keep people from sleeping through the night. This is the result of the constant postnasal mucus drainage from the sinuses, and mouth breathing subsequent to a stuffy nose. The dry air most of us breathe at night in our bedrooms can be very irritating. Once I've established that the sore throat is much worse first thing in the morning, the next step is to determine if there is any awareness of mucus draining down the back of the throat. In children, this drainage often results in bad breath. From that point I merely have to run through a checklist of the other potential sinus symptoms — mucus color, recent cold, fatigue, fever, etc. — to determine if this is sinusitis or something else. Most of these questions would be asked anyway as part of a thorough investigation of any sore throat.

Laryngitis

Laryngitis (hoarseness) is another common symptom of a sinus infection. It results from the same factors that cause sore throat, primarily postnasal mucus draining down into the larynx, causing irritation, inflammation and swelling of the vocal cords and the arytenoid cartilages.

Cough

I am sure that the chief complaints of cough and sore throat account for the bulk of the patients who come to a family doctor's office with a sinus infection. These are the symptoms that result in the greatest discomfort and the most loss of sleep. Unfortunately, they are also the symptoms that result in the highest number of misdiagnoses. A cough is often mistakenly thought to be bronchitis. Why? Because the cough of a sinusitis results from the same thing that causes the sore throat — yellow mucus draining down the back of the throat and continuing into the trachea or upper airway. Most physicians are aware that a productive (mucus-producing) cough that brings up a purulent or yellow mucus is often bronchitis. It isn't unusual to make that diagnosis in spite of hearing clear lungs with the stethoscope. So it's easy to understand this common mistake. But it's just as easy to ask a few simple questions to rule out bronchitis and rule in acute sinusitis.

The cough of a sinus infection in adults is invariably worse as soon as they lie down in bed at night. It isn't usually too bad during the day when they're upright. In children it tends to be more persistent throughout the day. We tend to swallow the postnasal mucus drainage, consciously or (usually) unconsciously, while we're up and about. This gets the mucus away from the trachea and into the stomach. (Swallowing the mucus can result in another not-uncommon symptom with sinus infections: gastrointestinal upset, i.e., abdominal discomfort and/or loose bowels. There may be two or three loosish bowel movements per day — not quite diarrhea, but a definite change in one's bowel pattern. This isn't nearly as common as the other symptoms I've mentioned, so I apologize for getting into another tract. Now, back to the cough.)

After asking about the timing of the cough, I usually want to know, "Does the cough feel like it's deep in your chest or does it feel more like a tickle in the back of your throat?" The latter, a drier cough, is much more typical of sinusitis, while the former, a wet mucusy cough, is more indicative of bronchitis. In the past year, I've noticed a definite increase in the number of patients who are infected in both the sinuses and the lungs simultaneously. Medicine calls this sinobronchitis. If the antibiotic treatments for sinusitis and bronchitis were the same, there would be no great necessity to differentiate between the two. However, this is not the case, and I believe it is valuable to be as specific as possible in a treatment program.

I began this chapter by describing acute sinusitis as an infection usually requiring medical attention. A visit to the doctor has a twofold purpose — to diagnose the problem and begin treating it. Ideally, there should also be a third objective — education, i.e., to teach the patient how to care for his sinuses so effectively that he can avoid any future office visits for the same problem. However, the feasibility of attaining this lofty goal in the midst of a busy practice has so far eluded me. It is from that frustration that the desire to write this book began.

As one can easily understand from reading this chapter, the recognition of acute sinusitis is not a simple matter, even for physicians. This chapter and the next should be referred to frequently. For those who are plagued with repeated sinus infections, you'll be surprised at how quickly and easily this new knowledge is absorbed.

CHRONIC SINUSITIS

For those of you who thought "acute" was no problem, perhaps I'll be able to challenge you with chronic sinusitis. This is the diagnosis believed by the National Center for Health Statistics to be the most common chronic condition in the United States. Yet, surprisingly enough, most people who have it couldn't tell you, and doctors have even more difficulty with this diagnosis than with acute sinusitis. The situation is similar to that of the hundreds of thousands of people who have high blood pressure and diabetes, which are other common chronic conditions, and are not aware of it. Although they may not be able to attach a label to it, what these sinus sufferers are very familiar with are mucus and tissues. Both have been a part of their daily lives for years and something most have just accepted. Doctors haven't paid much attention to chronic sinusitis because they don't consider it a significant disease, i.e., one that could shorten your life expectancy.

Chronic sinusitis is a persistent inflammation of the mucosal lining of the nose and sinus cavities. Cilia have become permanently damaged, making it more difficult for mucus to drain from the sinuses. It is not an infection. The diagnosis and recognition of this condition is made almost entirely on the basis of the patient's description of his condition — the medical history. An X-ray might reveal a thickened mucosa, which is not, however, necessarily diagnostic of this problem. A doctor's examination might show a deviated nasal septum or polyps in a small percentage of cases. These could have blocked the sinus opening, the ostia, contributing to the onset of chronic sinusitis.

However, for the vast majority of people, the condition began as a result of one or more episodes of acute sinusitis, repeated nasal allergies, or constant exposure to irritants such as smoke, pollution, fumes, etc. These factors can all leave the sinuses in a permanently damaged state.

What specific symptoms will help us in recognizing this chronic problem? They are generally mild and consist primarily of mucus drainage and head and nasal congestion. Most people wake up in the morning with clear or white mucus in the back of their throat and some mild nasal and/or head congestion. It isn't until after they've stepped out of a hot shower that they feel more "normal," their head is clear, and they're ready to face the day. During the day there is usually some nasal drainage, since they have an increased sensitivity to all of the factors I mentioned in Chapter 2 — smoke, pollution, dryness, fumes, etc. The more exposure to any one of these irritants, the more pronounced the symptoms will be. Headache and sinus or facial pain are not uncommon with heavy exposure to any of these things. A very reliable sign of a chronic sinusitis sufferer is that he or she never has a routine common cold. What starts out that way always results in an acute sinusitis. In fact, almost any infection, whether it begins as influenza, strep throat, gastroenteritis (vomiting and diarrhea), or a number of others, will often indirectly cause a sinus infection just by lowering their natural resistance.

Once again, it becomes quite clear that although I'm not describing a "serious" medical problem, it is very definitely a nagging nuisance type of condition. It affects us daily and has an impact on our ability to fully enjoy our lives. For most chronic sinus sufferers, there seems to be an increasing awareness of this problem.

Chapter 4

Treating Acute Sinusitis

TRADITIONAL MEDICAL METHODS

What does it mean to "treat" an ailment? It usually depends upon what the condition is. In some instances treatment implies cure, with the expectation that the problem will never recur. These treatments are most often surgical, e.g., appendicitis is treated with an appendectomy.

At other times, to treat means to improve symptoms in a condition that has no known cure. This could involve treating anything from cancer and AIDS to the common cold and sore throat. This category of treatment comprises the bulk of a physician's practice — almost 75 percent of all ailments fall into this treatment realm.

Acute sinusitis is a bacterial infection in one or more of the sinus cavities. The goal of treatment in this case is to kill the bacteria, open the blocked sinus duct, and restore the mucus/cilia cleansing system, while relieving all of the possible symptoms discussed in the last chapter. This type of treatment differs from the first two I mentioned. Acute sinusitis is an infection that does have a cure, but the chances of its recurring at some point, either months or years later, are very high.

Acute sinusitis is not a simple infection to treat, such as strep throat would be. The bacteria that cause the infection are rarely identified. An antibiotic is selected based upon the bacteria most likely to cause the infection (this is called an educated guess). The antibiotic is taken by mouth and absorbed into the bloodstream. But because of the relatively poor blood supply in the sinuses, it usually takes several days before the effect of the drug is felt, especially in adults. For this reason, strong antibiotics in relatively high dosages taken for long periods of time are often required to treat this infection.

The next objective is to open the blocked sinus duct and the ostium so that the infected mucus can drain from the sinus. The type of drug that best accomplishes the opening of the duct is a decongestant, since it shrinks the swollen mucous membrane. However, most decongestants also have a drying effect, especially if used in combination with an antihistamine. (Most commercial decongestants contain an antihistamine.) This drying will then thicken the mucus and prevent it from draining.

For those of you who expected the treatment to be easier than the diagnosis, I'm sorry to disappoint you. For the past few years my associates and I have continually been reevaluating and refining the medical treatment of acute sinusitis. It is an ongoing process, but it clearly seems to be getting more difficult to obtain a good result.

Antibiotics

The bacteria most often (about 75 percent of the time) responsible for causing sinus infections in both adults and children are *Streptococcus pneumoniae* and *Hemophilus influenzae*. Several other bacteria can cause the infection, but there is no single antibiotic that is effective against all of them and no simple laboratory test to determine which bacteria we're dealing with. Nasal cultures have been used for this purpose, but their reliability has never been widely accepted by the medical community.

For the past decade the first drug of choice has been ampicillin or its counterpart, amoxicillin. The dosage of ampicillin is 500 mg four times a day, or about every six hours, and for amoxicillin, 500 mg (250 mg in children) taken three times a day (every eight hours) for ten days. This is a routine first step, but it is a hefty dose of antibiotic! Adult patients are instructed that they will notice definite improvement and that the yellow mucus will start to clear in about four to five days. In children the response is usually faster, with fever, nasal drainage, and cough markedly reduced after about forty-eight hours. However, they are told to be sure to take the medicine for the entire ten days. Invariably, the sinusitis will return in full measure if they don't follow this instruction. (One of my associates routinely treats with amoxicillin for fourteen days instead of ten on the first go-round, which she believes decreases the number of treatment failures.)

Even if they do comply, about 5 to 10 percent of patients will return or call shortly after the ten days, still complaining of most of their same symptoms. Some will report that they felt much better while on the antibiotic, but that as soon as they stopped, the symptoms recurred. Others will tell me they experienced no improvement whatsoever, and usually in a tone of voice that conveys the very clear message, "You'd better get rid of this infection real fast." These are not my most pleasant patients. Nor should they be. They've usually had the sinusitis for at least three weeks and have now made their second visit to the doctor.

With my second attempt at treatment, I'll almost always choose a different antibiotic. The second-choice antibiotics have a bit broader spectrum of efficacy than amoxicillin; all of them are more expensive. Table 1 lists both amoxicillin and the second-step drugs that are

Table 1.
ANTIBIOTICS FOR ACUTE SINUSITIS

Brand Name & Quantity	Generic Equivalent	Strength/Average Dose	Adults (12 + yr.) or Children	Average Price
	Amoxicillin Capsules #30	1) 250 mg 1 3X/day 2) 500 mg for 10 days	1) children 2) adults	1) $5 2) $7
	Amoxicillin Suspension 150 cc	250 mg 5cc (1 tsp.) 3X/dX10 d	children	$6
Ceclor Capsules 1) #20; 2) #30		250 mg 1) 1 2X/dX10 d 2) 3X/dX10 d	adults	1) $27 2) $40
Ceclor Suspension 150 cc		250 mg 5 cc 3X/dX10 d	children	$36
Bactrim DS #20 or Septra DS	Trimethoprim- Sulfamethoxazole	1 2X/da. X 10 d	adults	$25 $11 (generic)
Bactrim Suspension 200 cc	Trimethoprim- Sulfamethoxazole	10 cc (2 tsp) 2X/dX10 d	children	$14 $6 (generic)
Vibramycin or Vibra-Tabs #20	Doxycycline	100 mg 1 2X/dX10 d	adults	$44 $8 (generic)
Pediazole Suspension 200 cc		5 cc 4X/d X 10 d	children	$24

commonly used for the treatment of acute sinusitis. The one I use most often is Ceclor (250 mg). It has been, in my practice, the most reliable with the least side effects (about 1 to 2 percent of patients develop a severe skin rash). Unfortunately, it is also the most expensive. Many physicians report excellent results with the others, as well. The latest antibiotic being used, Ceftin, is reported to be extremely effective for sinusitis.

In a few difficult-to-treat patients, the infection returns even after these heavier antibiotics. These patients I will usually treat for up to fourteen days and begin *gradually* tapering their dose from three capsules a day (with Ceclor) to one capsule a day over the last five days. With some of them, I've even had to increase the strength of the Ceclor to 500 mg. At three capsules a day for two weeks, this can be close to a $100 prescription! Fortunately, these cases are still very infrequent. But when they do occur, and I'm not dealing with a smoker, then it is appropriate to obtain an X-ray to see if there is a structural problem obstructing the sinus.

Decongestants

The decongestants are specifically used to open the ostia and sinus ducts while relieving the symptoms of head and nasal congestion, facial pain, and to some extent, sore throat and cough.

As I've already mentioned, the challenge of using a decongestant in the treatment of acute sinusitis is to find one whose benefits outweigh the side effects. Decongestants are readily available in many familiar over-the-counter products, e.g., Dristan, Contac, Allerest, Drixoral, Actifed, Dimetapp, Triaminicin, and a host of other "cold remedies." However, every one of these has an antihistamine in combination with the decongestant. This is also true of Sinutab and many other "sinus remedies." Given the drying effect of antihistamines and the subsequent thickening of the mucus as a result of this drying, I'm convinced they do more harm than good. They're fine if all you're trying to treat is a cold. But in many instances, I believe they've actually helped a cold progress into a sinus infection. So, if you have a history of sinus problems, I would advise you never to take an antihistamine. If you're not sure about the ingredients of a decongestant, ask the pharmacist.

Now that it's clear what not to take, I'll be more specific on what few products there are that would be helpful. The best one is a prescription drug called Entex.* I believe Entex is the best because it contains not only two decongestants, phenylephrine and phenylpropanolamine ("Entex" is much easier to remember), but also a mucus-thinning agent as well — guaifenisen. It comes in both capsules and liquid, so it can be used by both adults and children. It's meant to be taken several times (usually three) a day, and its effect lasts from four to six hours. Entex should not be used by anyone with high blood pressure. The most common side effect in adults is that it can keep them awake at night. Omitting the bedtime dose will eliminate this side effect. Some

---

* Recently, there's been a competitor — Duragest. It's chemically identical to Entex, with a different brand name.

younger children experience the opposite side effect — drowsiness. Entex also comes in another form, called Entex-LA, a tablet that lasts for ten to twelve hours. I don't prescribe this as often as plain Entex, since it isn't as strong. It contains only one decongestant.

I usually don't insist that patients with acute sinusitis take Entex as regularly as I do the antibiotic, or for the entire ten-day course. I tell them to take it regularly for the first four to five days, then gradually taper off. If they're still experiencing head and sinus congestion, then they should continue with it. Due to the poor air quality and pressure changes experienced on airplanes, I also frequently take Entex during air travel, approximately two hours prior to the scheduled landing time. However, if the flight can be avoided while one still has an active sinus infection, it is advisable to postpone it.

Another prescription drug that works well is Respaire-SR. It only comes in a long-acting (twelve-hour) form. It can also cause insomnia, but it can be used by those with high blood pressure.

An over-the-counter alternative for those with extreme head and nasal congestion and/or sinus pain is nasal decongestant spray. There are several twelve-hour varieties from which to choose. These should be used with great caution and only for a day or two. They can easily become addictive! They produce what is called a rebound effect, which means that as their decongestant effect wears off and the head and nasal congestion return, the feeling of stuffiness is worse than it was before using the spray. This elicits a strong desire to spray again, and so on. Be careful with these! If you've been using a spray regularly and are unable to stop, you'll probably need some help. I would consult with your physician and tell him honestly what's been happening. I've had a high success rate in helping patients to break this habit by using the following regimen:

— Throw away the nasal spray.

— Medrol (generic = methylprednisolone) dosepak 4 mg; this is a tapered dose of cortisone over a six-day period and is a prescription drug.

— Entex — a prescription for forty capsules to be taken in a tapered (one 3 times/day X 7 days; then one 2 times/day X 7 days; followed by one daily (before bed) X 7 days dose over three weeks.

— Moisture — includes saline nasal spray, ultrasonic humidifier, and steaming in the bathroom (refer to the "Moisture" section in this chapter).

Remember that it is extremely difficult to have healthy sinuses with continued use of a decongestant nasal spray.

Several other decongestants are found in combination with cough suppressants, expectorants, and analgesics, which I will mention later with respect to coughing. If you ever find yourself desperately congested and without a prescription for Entex, the following are all acceptable over-the-counter alternatives: Robitussin-PE, Naldecon-EX, Sine-Aid, Tylenol Sinus, Sinutab II, Sine-Off, and Sudafed. The first two have the least drying effect, and all of those that have "Sin" in their name contain the pain reliever acetaminophen in combination with a decongestant.

Analgesics (Pain Relievers)

To relieve the frequent symptoms of headache, facial pain, and sore throat, I recommend the over-the-counter pain relievers Advil or Nuprin. Both contain ibuprofen, which not only relieves pain, but also reduces inflammation. To some extent, it can lower a fever. They are dispensed in 200-mg tablets, and it is safe (for adults) to take three or even four of them at a time if the pain is especially severe. This dosage should usually be taken with food, especially if there is a history of stomach ulcers.

Aspirin has the same effects as ibuprofen but isn't as strong. Tylenol and other acetaminophen-containing products are simply analgesics, with no effect upon the inflamed sinuses. However, if lowering a fever is the primary objective, then both aspirin and Tylenol would be better choices. Any acetaminophen-containing product is the drug of choice for children.

Moisture

Moisture helps to empty the sinus of its thick infected mucus and in doing so aids in restoring normal cilial function. As it does this, it also relieves nasal and head congestion, headache, sinus pain, and sore throat. Warm, moist air is best, and the easiest place to get it is in the bathroom. Simply close the door and window and turn on the hot water of the shower to create steam. Then you have the choice of either getting in the shower (after adjusting the temperature, of course) or just sitting and relaxing in the steam until you run out of hot water. Remember to try and make a conscious effort to breathe through your nose, thereby getting the moisture where it will do the most good. Hot towels applied over the face can also be helpful.

Since most of us do not have an endless supply of hot water in our homes, making a steam room of your bathroom can only be done two or three times a day. What about the rest of the time? If you've decided to stay home from work, your best alternative for moist air is a steam humidifier placed by your bed, with the bedroom door and windows closed. A recent study showed that the more popular ultrasonic humidifiers give off a significant amount of mineral particles which may make life harder for your sinuses. Running them on distilled or filtered water and keeping the door or window open will improve this situation, but steam humidifiers are still the cleanest of all. Since the water is boiled, the minerals never leave the machine. Whether you're home or not during the day, it should be used every night while you're treating the sinus infection. The moisture is very helpful in relieving both the cough and sore throat during the night.

Another simple method for obtaining moisture (this assumes your environment is relatively dry, as indoor air tends to be during the winter months in most parts of the United States), is to use a salt water (saline) nasal spray. There are several commercial products available in many pharmacies, e.g., Salinex, Ayr, or Ocean spray. You can also make your own by mixing a teaspoon of salt in a 16-ounce (1-pint) glass of lukewarm water and dispensing from a spray bottle. You should spray in each nostril while pinching off the other nostril and simultaneously inhaling through your nose. This can be done as often as you'd like throughout the day. It's non-addicting and has no negative side effects that I'm aware of, except for the curious looks you'll get from those wanting to know what in the world you're doing.

A more effective way of moisturizing, but more importantly, irrigating, is a saline irrigation. This procedure can result in dramatic relief from pain. The reduction of pressure in the sinus also improves blood flow. The salt water sprays that I just mentioned also irrigate, i.e., wash out mucus, bacteria, dust particles, etc., while reducing swelling in the nasal passages. But they don't do it as well as the following methods, which should be used three to four times a day.

Make the irrigating (saline) solution fresh each day in one cup of lukewarm tap water. Add ¼ to ½ teaspoon of table salt and a tiny pinch of baking soda, making the solution close to normal body fluid salinity and pH. Use the full cup of saline solution for each irrigation, and irrigate with the head inclined over the sink but in an upright position. Always blow the nose *very* gently after irrigating.

Method 1. Completely fill a large all-rubber ear syringe (available at most pharmacies) with saline solution. Lean way over sink, and pinch one nostril closed. Insert syringe tip just inside the open nostril, pinching nostril around tip. *Gently* squeeze bulb and release several times to swish solution around inside the nose. The solution will run out both nostrils and may also run out the mouth. Repeat for each nostril until one cup of saline solution is used.

Method 2. Pour saline solution into palm of hand, and sniff solution up the nose, one nostril at a time. Spit out solution and blow the nose very lightly afterwards.

Method 3. Use angled nasal irrigator attachment (available at some pharmacies) on a Water Pik appliance. Set Water Pik at lowest possible pressure and insert irrigator tip just inside nostril, pinching nostril to seal. Irrigate with mouth open, allowing fluid to drain out either mouth or nose.

Method 4. For very small children, irrigate with ten to twenty drops of saline solution per nostril from an eyedropper.

If you are using a decongestant nasal spray, use it only AFTER the salt water nasal irrigations.

This method obviously requires more effort than the saline nasal sprays, but many patients have commented on how helpful it has been.

Another solution which has been extremely effective in irrigation is called Alkalol. It is a mucus solvent and cleaner, and can be used with the saline solution in a 1:1 ratio (½ saline, ½ Alkalol) with all of the above methods. You'll probably have to ask your pharmacist to order it for you because it is not usually available. It's very inexpensive.

Cough Suppressants

If a patient's chief complaint is a cough that's not allowing him to sleep, I'll withhold his bedtime dose of Entex and use instead a powerful cough suppressant. My first choice is usually Donatussin DC, which combines the most effective cough suppressant, hydrocodone, with a decongestant and an expectorant. Another good combination drug is Naldecon-CX, which has codeine as its cough suppressant. These are both prescription drugs that can cause drowsiness. That's why I rarely recommend them for daytime use. Besides, these people are already tired from having a sinus infection. They don't need any additional sedation.

During the day, if a cough suppressant is indicated, especially in children, there are several similar over-the-counter combination drugs from which to choose. They can be taken by both adults and children. The brand names are as follows: Sudafed cough syrup, Naldecon-DX, Robitussin-CF, Vicks Formula 44M and 44D, Novahistine DMX, and Dorcol. They all have the same cough suppressant, dextromethorphan, which is non-sedating. They each also have an expectorant to thin the mucus, as well as a decongestant. They would be used instead of Entex.

Hydration and Bed Rest

How often have you heard the advice, "Drink lots of liquids and stay in bed"? Even with acute sinusitis it still holds true. I recommend at least doubling your normal fluid intake with primarily water and fruit juices. Avoid ice-cold drinks and anything with caffeine or alcohol.

As for resting, try to listen to your body and not push yourself. You don't literally have to stay in bed, but do as much resting as possible during the first five to seven days of treatment.

The office policy that I have been using for the

treatment of sinus infections in a previously seen sinus patient is to phone in prescriptions for the antibiotic and decongestant upon their request. Doctors are taught that the practice of "good medicine" does not permit them to prescribe antibiotics without first seeing the patient. This is a valid principle and works well in most instances. However, in my practice, I and my four associates agreed to this exception: If we have seen a patient at least once with acute sinusitis, and within the next two years he or she calls to report another sinus infection and would like a prescription phoned in to the pharmacy, then we will do it. This assumes that we have spent some time educating that patient about sinusitis in our office. I hope that most of you are able to find a physician who will be similarly understanding with your sinus condition. Don't be discouraged if you can't find one at first; there are others. I realize that some of you, after reading to this point, will feel as if you know more about your own sinuses than the doctor. You may be right, but I strongly advocate establishing a relationship with a physician if you'd like to pursue the medically recommended "antibiotic route" that I've described. Should you opt not to enter the medical system, everything I've described in this chapter is still available to you with the exception of the antibiotic, Entex, and a strong cough suppressant.

HOLISTIC METHODS

Holistic medicine has a much broader conception of a human being than traditional medicine. It views a patient as body, mind, emotions, and spirit, rather than merely a body with a broken or malfunctioning part. This approach recognizes that the integrity and balance of the whole (all four components) is the key to health and well-being. "Dis-ease" results from stress in one or more of the four aspects of an individual, with a subsequent loss of balance, integration, and harmony in the whole being. Although this imbalance is most clearly manifested in the physical component, the whole person is affected. Holistic medicine looks at the doctor/patient relationship as a partnership working toward the goal of the patient ultimately learning to heal him/herself.

The holistic methods that I'll briefly discuss here are homeopathy, reflexology, finger acupressure, Chinese medicine, and spiritual healing. Although none of these modalities has been scientifically proven, I know that each of them can be effective in treating sinusitis, both acute and chronic.

The critical factor in the success of these methods (or any method) is the patient's belief that it can succeed. In our society most of us believe that medical science is our only acceptable option for the treatment of not only acute sinusitis but most other physical ailments as well. Therefore, prior to attempting a holistic approach, this belief must be modified, so that it is at least possible for this alternative method to work.

The *homeopathic* approach utilizes herbs — the Earth's "natural medicines." Garlic and onions are considered to be our most powerful natural antibiotics. In the treatment of acute sinusitis, they are used liberally in capsule form or eaten as a part of the diet. Two garlic capsules (10 minums) can be taken three times a day. Some vitamin stores now carry a combination garlic/onion tablet, four of which should be taken three times a day for a sinus infection. The homeopathic diet also eliminates all sugar and milk products and emphasizes the need for lots of parsley, celery, and spinach to replenish the chlorophyll that the infection has depleted. Chlorophyll capsules are available at health food stores and can be taken in liberal doses. To help revitalize the body's immune system, the following salt capsules are recommended: Kal Mur #5 (KCl), Nat Mur #9 (NaCl), and Ferr Phos #4 (FePh). These, too, can be purchased at most health food stores. They should be taken at least six times a day. Vitamin C, 1000 mg, taken three times a day, then gradually tapered over several days, also helps to fight the infection. Other herbs that I've found to be effective are Nature's Way HAS and goldenseal root.

To open the sinuses and assist in mucus drainage, the following maneuvers are used: (1) with the index finger and thumb over the bridge of the nose between the eyebrows, pinch hard; and (2) with both index fingers by the side of the nose, massage (Figure F). Both of these should be performed for four to five seconds, either sitting or lying down. The pressure should be applied hard enough to cause some discomfort. These procedures can be repeated several times a day; they come under the heading of *finger acupressure.*

There are also points on both the toes and hands (Figure G) where pressure should be applied with your fingers or the eraser part of a pencil for several seconds and with enough pressure to cause some discomfort. These are part of the technique of *reflexology.*

There are two parts of the colon (large bowel) whose malfunctioning is associated with sinus infections — the ileocecal and transverse colon. To treat the sinus, maneuvers are performed on both of these areas of the bowel. The ileocecal area is approximately midway along an imaginary line drawn between the crest or uppermost part of the pelvis (hip bone) and the navel. This area is jabbed with the fingertips of your right hand and the hand is rotated in a clockwise, then counterclockwise motion while the fingertips are still touching the abdomen. For the transverse colon, a colon cleanse is recommended. This consists of several

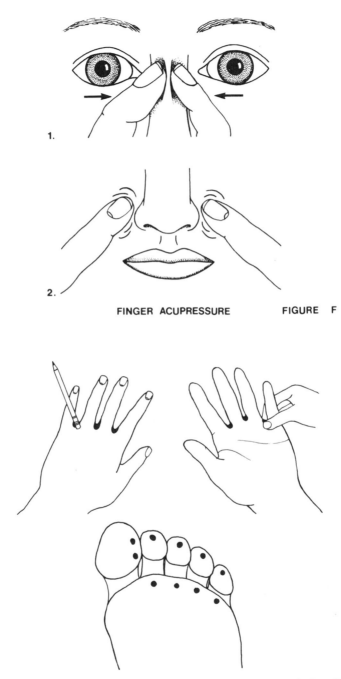

FINGER ACUPRESSURE   FIGURE F

REFLEXOLOGY   FIGURE G

ingredients, taken three times a day, which can be purchased at health food stores. There are several brand names, e.g., Colon #8, ABC by Aerobic, or Colon Cleanse.

Chinese medicine attempts to balance the body's vital energy, called *qi* (pronounced *chee*). It involves herbs, diet, and acupuncture. You will need to find a practitioner of this art. Sinus infections are believed to result from a problem in the lungs, spleen, and liver.

The herbal regimen used to treat acute sinusitis consists of the following:
— Ching-Pi-Tang (Pueraria Nasal Combination) — contains thirteen herbs
— Bi Yan tablets — consists of twelve herbs
— Nasal Oil — drops
— White Flower Oil

Acupuncture might require anywhere from one to four sessions, with the needles being primarily around the sinuses. These sessions last from thirty minutes to an hour and are not expensive. In a case of severe illness with the infection, the patient might visit the acupuncturist three times within a week.

The dietary recommendations made by Chinese medicine for sinusitis stress the following: warm foods — avoid cold or raw vegetables and fruits; lots of hot soups, herbal teas, stews, chili, hot cereals (oatmeal), and other grains — brown rice, buckwheat, wheat, and rye; chicken, fish, and root vegetables (warm) — carrots, potatoes, cabbage; no dairy products. These are reasonable dietary guidelines to adhere to for general good health.

Spiritual healing is a holistic approach which might also be called "God's healing." It is based upon the understanding that God is love, and that unconditional love and God are synonymous terms. Its purpose is to produce a heightened state of awareness of love in each of the four components of a human being. This is accomplished through the daily practice of techniques which help the individual determine what feels most like love to him or her. Since each of us is a unique being, no two people will practice spiritual healing in exactly the same way.

As with any method of holistic medicine it is believed that stress is the cause of dis-ease. In Louise Hay's book, *You Can Heal Your Life* (an excellent guide to spiritual healing), she asserts that the stressor causing acute sinusitis is irritation with one person, someone close. A new thought pattern that helps to overcome this problem can be established through the use of affirmations. These are positive statements that should be repeated verbally and/or written down as many times as possible. The basic affirmation for sinusitis is as follows: "I declare peace and harmony indwell me and surround me at all times. All is well." Another one which should be repeated often is, "My sinuses are now completely healed." You should try to make an affirmation personal, and it should not contain any negative words. Affirmations can be used to change any belief.

In addition to affirmations, the following are only a few of the many techniques that could be incorporated into your daily life:

— a healthy diet (refer to "Diet" in Chapter 6)
— aerobic exercise: walking, hiking, jogging, cycling, swimming (use nose plugs in a chlorinated pool), rowing, low-impact aerobics, dance, cross-country skiing; maintain a pulse rate of 220 minus your age x 70 to 80% (use 60% or less during the early stages of a sinus infection); maintain this rate for a minimum of 20 minutes at least 3 times a week.
— forgiveness: remember that you and everyone else are always doing the best they can; say the affirmations, "I am always doing the best I can. There are

no mistakes.''
— meditation or any form of conscious breathing or breathing exercise, several times (3 or 4)/day for a few minutes; try to draw the inhale gently but deeply into the chest, then simply relax on the exhale, letting the breath flow out freely
— mental imagery: can be done while meditating; create a mental picture which symbolizes for you a healing sinus
— healing or loving touch: touch your face, cheeks, and forehead (sinuses) in as compassionate and loving a manner as you can; someone else who loves you could also do this for you; remember to be in a relaxed position while focusing on breathing and feelings of love
— acknowledge and express feelings: if there is no one to talk to, then express the feelings out loud to yourself, especially those of fear and anger
— psalms: read three psalms daily; 121 in the morning, 91 after work and 23 before bed
— prayer: use any prayer that you're comfortable with and repeat it twice daily, after arising and before bed.

By listening to your intuition, acknowledging your feelings, and trusting your choices, you will be able to become a skilled practitioner in the art of spiritual healing.

I've presented only a few of the many alternatives that are available to treat acute sinusitis. I would suggest trying more than one; perhaps a combination of several of the methods. My point in presenting these alternatives is merely to demonstrate that there are, in fact, other ways of treating acute sinusitis. Most Americans will likely choose the ease, simplicity, and familiarity of taking medication. However, a growing number of people are dissatisfied with the traditional medical approach. For them and anyone else looking for something "new" (most of these holistic alternatives are actually ancient forms of healing), there are many options available. All that's required is an open mind and the belief that "maybe it's possible!"

Chapter 5

When Sinusitis Coexists with Other Medical Conditions

It is not uncommon for acute sinusitis to coexist with other conditions that also affect the respiratory tract. In almost every instance when this occurs, it is the accompanying problem, not the sinus infection, that is most apparent to both physician and patient. Two of these problems — the common cold and nasal allergies — precede the onset of acute sinusitis, while the others occur subsequent to the sinus infection.

The Common Cold

This is the most frequent condition concomitant with sinusitis. Since it has been discussed from different perspectives in Chapters 2, 3, and 4, there is little left to say. I will, however, remind you that if you're at all suspicious of a sinus infection, or you're at high risk for getting one, then avoid taking antihistamines. Every cold can be treated in the same way that I recommended for acute sinusitis, with the exception of the antibiotic. If the sinus infection is present along with the cold, it should become obvious in seven to ten days.

Acute Otitis Media (Middle Ear Infection)

This is quite commonly seen in children, and very often in conjunction with acute sinusitis. The bacteria that cause this infection are identical to those responsible for sinus infections. The position and anatomy of the eustachian tube, which drains the middle ear space, helps to create the simultaneous infections. I once heard an ENT physician say that any time you see an adult with otitis media, that person always has an underlying acute sinusitis.

When otitis media is present, sinusitis is usually ignored or not even recognized. Most of these patients are extremely uncomfortable with ear pain, and that becomes the focus of attention for both doctor and patient. Young children will also usually have a significant (above 101° F) fever. The treatment of otitis media can be exactly the same as that of acute sinusitis, so that even if the diagnosis of sinusitis is missed, the sinus infection usually will get better anyway. In adults with otitis media, however, I would recommend more regular use of Entex than I would for children, and for a longer period of time than I would with sinusitis (three times a day for at least ten days). This is because adults with middle ear infections routinely complain of "stuffiness" in their ears long after the pain has gone, often for two to three weeks.

Many young children have repeated episodes of acute otitis media, as often as four or five times within a year. Family physicians and pediatricians are very familiar with this kind of patient. What is probably happening with most of them is that each cold they get quickly becomes a sinus infection, which then subsequently causes the ear infection. Since the average number of colds per year in young kids can be as great as six, that can occasion lots of visits to the doctor or an emergency room (ear infections often begin at night). Many of these pediatric patients will eventually require surgery (involving the placement of tubes through the eardrums).

Allergic Rhinitis (Nasal Allergy)

When allergies accompany sinusitis, or the patient suffering from allergy symptoms is known to have a history of sinus infections, the problem becomes one of the more challenging ones in medicine. Since allergy results in swelling and inflammation of the nasal mucous membrane and blockage of the sinus ducts, it is important to be able to treat these symptoms without creating a sinus infection. An acute flare-up of a runny nose and cough or difficulty controlling nasal congestion with the usual allergy therapy may signal the presence of a sinus infection.

Most people with seasonal nasal allergy, also known as hay fever, rely upon over-the-counter medications for relief. Many of these I mentioned in Chapter 4, e.g., Dristan, Contac, Allerest, Drixoral, Actifed, Dimetapp, Triaminicin, and Sudafed-Plus. They are helpful primarily because of the antihistamine that they all contain, in addition to a decongestant. Chlortrimeton is another popular one, but without a decongestant. Antihistamines are wonderful drugs for the treatment of allergies, although they do cause drowsiness. But as you may recall, they're terrible for the person with weak sinuses or one who already has a sinus infection since they cause increased viscosity or thickening of the mucus.

If you have an allergy in addition to sinusitis, then you should try to treat your allergy without the use of antihistamines. Both Nasalcrom spray and the cortisone sprays — Beconase, Vancenase, and Nasalide — are all very effective for the treatment of nasal allergy. They work even better if used subsequent to nasal irrigation (described in the "Moisture" section of Chapter 4). This will remove the mucus secretions so the spray won't sit on the mucus but will directly hit the lining of the nose. The irrigation will remove allergens (pollen) as well. In the case of a seasonal allergy sufferer, the spray should be used throughout the season. Since the majority of people with hay fever are reacting to either tree pollen (April/May), grasses (May/June), or weeds (August/September), they should use the spray on a daily basis for at least a month. This recommendation applies to all those with allergy symptoms having a history of sinus infections. They'll not only obtain effective relief for their symptoms, but likely will also avoid both the acute sinusitis and the drowsiness. If someone already has an acute sinusitis along with the hay fever, which can be a very difficult diagnosis to make, the patient should use the regular sinusitis treatment regimen in addition to Nasalcrom or the cortisone spray. Some of these people are so uncomfortable that I'll add a short course of cortisone tablets.

Bronchitis and Pneumonia

I've already described in Chapter 3 the condition called sinobronchitis, i.e., sinusitis coexisting with bronchitis. It is being seen with greater frequency and is also not a simple diagnosis to make. The cough is usually the primary complaint. It is a persistent (day and night), deep, wet, and mucusy (yellow) cough, often found in smokers. The usual symptoms of sinusitis are also present. Needless to say, these people seem more ill than the typical acute sinusitis patient.

Worse yet are those whose bronchitis has turned into pneumonia, which is simply a more severe lung infection than the bronchitis. These patients are quite sick with a bad cough and often fever and chills.

Both of these lung infections can usually be diagnosed by listening to the lungs with a stethoscope; pneumonia can be confirmed with a chest X-ray. When a sinus infection is also present, it most likely will have preceded these lung conditions and probably created them with the postnasal drainage of infected mucus into the lungs.

Following the diagnosis, the next step lies in selecting an antibiotic that will cure both infections. It will be difficult to get rid of the infection in the lungs if the sinusitis is still present. It is for this reason that I will not choose erythromycin to start treatment. Although it may be the best choice for the lungs, I have seen many instances in which it was ineffective in treating a sinus infection. I'll usually begin with doxycycline, and if significant improvement is not evident in four to five days, I'll then add erythromycin. The rest of the treatment program is the same as it is for sinusitis, with the addition of postural drainage techniques to help clear the lungs of infection.

Asthma

This is another disease of the lungs which is very much affected by sinusitis. In a study published in 1987 by the National Jewish Center for Immunology and Respiratory Medicine in Denver, a national research center for asthma and other respiratory diseases, it was noted that half of the patients in the study with mild or severe asthma had sinus abnormalities on X-ray. It was also reported that sinus treatment of asthmatic children with moderate to severe sinus abnormalities may improve the course of their asthma. The study made reference to a report completed in 1925 that postulated four mechanisms that might explain how sinus disease could cause asthma. Those conclusions were not substantially different from the ones made in the 1987 study. Two of these mechanisms are quite similar to what was mentioned in Chapter 3 with respect to the symptoms of cough, sore throat, and laryngitis. They are (1) postnasal drip of mucus into the lower airways, which either directly alters the airways' reactivity or causes the airways' inflammation, and (2) mouth breathing of cold and/or dry air due to nasal obstruction, which elicits asthma by increasing heat and water loss in the lower airways.

The National Jewish Center treats primarily asthmatics who are poorly controlled and/or steroid (cortisone) dependent. (Ironically, the hospital sits in one of the highest air pollution locations in the entire city.) Their study linking sinus disease to asthma described many asthmatics who improved dramatically and were able to decrease their steroid requirements following treatment of their sinusitis. If this holds true for the worst asthmatics, then it should also apply to anyone with mild to moderate asthma who is experiencing a flare-up or an exacerbation of their condition. If an obvious cause for the asthmatic episode is not present, e.g., common cold, allergy, exercise, etc., and the wheezing can't be controlled with the usual medication, then think of the possibility of a sinus infection.

That is also the message for the other conditions described in this chapter. I am trying to instill a greater level of awareness of the existence of sinusitis. Not only can the sinus infection be subtle in its presentation, but when it accompanies these other conditions, it can have a profound impact on the course of the illness.

Chapter 6

Treating Chronic Sinusitis

Since chronic sinusitis is considered to be an incurable condition, the treatment program can only alleviate symptoms and minimize the risk of future sinus infections while improving the quality of life. This will require a commitment on the part of the chronic sinus sufferer to incorporate new practices into his lifestyle.

The most important element in attaining these goals is a heightened awareness of all the factors that make sinuses worse: the common cold; air pollution; cigarettes; hot, dry, and cold air; fumes; allergies; and emotional stress. Since most of these factors have something to do with air quality, the primary objective of any treatment program must involve modifying and somehow enhancing the air in our environment.

I'm sure it's obvious to many readers at this point that living in a place having warm, moist, and clean air with cigarette smoking prohibited is close to ideal. You would be absolutely right! But go try to find such a place.

For Americans, obviously some regions are better than others. The entire West Coast, with the distinct exception of the Los Angeles area, is probably the best. Here you have prevailing westerly winds blowing in from the Pacific Ocean. The air is not only extremely clean, its moisture content is quite pleasant, unlike the uncomfortable humidity experienced in many other parts of the country. The air temperatures also tend to be moderate, with infrequent extremes. I read an article several years ago in *Outside* magazine that ranked San Juan County, outside of Seattle, as the most livable county in America. Marin County, across the Golden Gate Bridge from San Francisco, was said to have the most ideal climate of any county in the United States. Florida, the southeastern states, the Gulf Coast, and southern Texas are also good places to investigate. I realize there are many people who live in these areas who do have sinus problems. Remember that the common cold, the pollens that trigger nasal allergies, occupational risks, and emotional stress have not been eliminated from these areas.

For those of you who would like to remain in your present home, and it isn't located in any of these optimum areas, let's get down to business. What can you do on a daily basis to improve your sinus condition?

Attempting to modify the outdoor air on an individual basis will be an uphill struggle. Not until the air quality reaches crisis proportions will any significant changes be made. We're almost there, and that point will surely be reached within the next decade. But it will then require a massive cooperative effort on the part of entire communities to effect a substantial improvement in our air pollution.

Air Cleaners

You have a much better chance of improving the *indoor* air than the outdoor air. Here you have a closed and more controlled environment. The best method I've found for cleaning the air in your home is an electrostatic air cleaner attached to the furnace in a forced-hot-air heating system. The one I have was purchased at Sears for about $600. It works quite well and is certainly preferable to dusting your entire home each day.

There are other air cleaners that can do individual

rooms, and some of these are effective in trapping pollen. A rather inexpensive (about $100) and handy gadget that also cleans each room is a negative ion generator. This small device quietly produces negative ions (charged particles) that attract dust, pollen, and other particles in the air and cause them to drop to the floor or on objects in the room. When using a room air cleaner make sure the bedroom (assuming this is the most practical room to keep clean) door and windows are closed. Turn it on several hours before you plan to go to bed. One other note on clean air — be sure to change the filter on the furnace frequently (monthly during the winter).

Decongestants

Have Entex available and use it as needed, but sparingly. There may be situations where you can anticipate that you'll experience congestion, e.g., a smoke-filled room, or a change in altitude if you're flying or even driving to a different elevation. Any instance where you are reasonably sure you'll have significant head and/or nasal congestion, I'd recommend using Entex preventively.

For more information about decongestants, please refer to that section in Chapter 4.

Moisture

Everything I mentioned in Chapter 4 about moisture will also apply to the care of chronic sinusitis.

A hot, steamy shower is an excellent way to start the day. It opens the nasal passages, ostia, and sinus ducts and allows the mucus to drain.

A steam humidifier should be placed by the side of the bed and used every night, especially during the winter months. In a particularly arid climate such as Denver's, it's helpful to use it during the summer months too.

I also recommend having a humidifier attached to the furnace. Such attachments will help improve the moisture content in the whole house, although they are not as effective for individual rooms as the steam humidifiers. They cost about $200. Remember to keep the humidifiers clean, for they can grow both mold and fungus.

An innovative but much more expensive method of creating more moisture in the home is an indoor hot tub or spa. Its feasibility will depend upon available space and, more importantly, available funds. The total cost could be as much as $4000. An open or spacious configuration of the home will optimize a hot tub's potential as a humidifier. It's also lots of fun and will certainly add another dimension to your life.

A saline spray bottle should become a part of your wardrobe. It's good for both humidity and irrigation and helps to minimize the effects of cigarette smoke, air pollution, fumes, and hot and dry air. It can also decrease the incidence of colds by flushing out viruses. Use it as often as you'd like; you can't overdo it. Please refer to the "Moisture" section of Chapter 4 for any additional explanation.

Peppermint Oil

This is something else that seems to help. I put a very small amount (one drop is enough) on my fingertip, then wipe it around the *outside* of both nostrils. The oil, which acts as a stimulant, improves circulation to the nasal and sinus mucous membranes. This enhances the effect of the clean and moist air. I like to spray my nose with the saline spray or stand in front of the humidifier and then apply the peppermint oil. It feels wonderful! Eucalyptus oil has a similar effect. These oils can be purchased at most health food stores and even some pharmacies. The use of peppermint oil can become a daily practice and can be applied as often as you'd like. The greatest limit to its frequent use may be the possible complaints of family or coworkers about its odor. Personally, I think it smells great!

Vitamins

Although most physicians have discounted Nobel Prize winner Linus Pauling's work with regard to Vitamin C and the common cold, there is ample empirical evidence attesting to its value. For those willing to take a "chance," I recommend a daily dose of 3000 mg (for children, 750 mg) of Vitamin C with rose hips. It can be purchased in 1000-mg tablets, and one tablet should be taken with each meal. Vitamin C will help to prevent colds by bolstering the body's immune system. It is also reputed to have a beneficial effect upon the mucous membrane of the nose and sinuses, and there are those who believe it helps to prevent cancer. Even if it accomplishes none of these things, the risk of taking this dose of Vitamin C is negligible. Even though there is no good method of proving whether it has prevented any colds, I have seen its benefit in greatly reducing the symptoms and severity of a cold.

At the first sign of a cold, increase the amount of Vitamin C to 12,000 mg. This should be the total daily dose for day one of the cold. On the second day, reduce the amount to 10,000 mg, and continue tapering to 8000 mg, 6000 mg, 4000 mg, then back to 3000 mg on the sixth day. For children, I would use about one-quarter of these adult dosages. The total daily amount should be taken in three divided doses with meals. The most obvious side effect of all of this Vitamin C, other than a milder cold, will be quite similar to what one would experience following a meal of beans. Lots of flatulence! But this is a small price to pay for not only minimizing the cold but also decreasing the chances of developing a subsequent sinus infection. If acute sinusitis can be avoided, then there will be less damage to the mucous membrane and the chronic sinusitis will ultimately be less severe.

I also recommend a daily multivitamin. The best one I've found is called Magna II, made by Radiance. It has a high dosage of everything, especially the B vitamins, which are also good for the sinuses.

For the past several years, I've taken one garlic capsule (dosage 10 minums) two or three times a day with meals. With its potential value as a natural antibiotic, I decided it would be worthwhile to include as part of my daily vitamin regimen.

Diet

More important than the vitamin supplements is a well-balanced diet. It should be high in fruits, vegetables, and whole grains (e.g., wheat, brown rice, buckwheat, oats, rye, corn meal, barley, couscous, and bulghur), and especially low in milk and dairy products and anything with preservatives. Good sources of protein are fish, turkey, chicken, and tofu. Remember to make an effort to drink lots (four to six glasses) of clean, i.e., bottled, water every day. What I'm suggesting is a healthy diet, one that would be beneficial for anyone, with or without sinus problems. However, the person with chronic sinusitis has a physical weakness, and an effective way to strengthen the body is to improve the quality of the diet.

Exercise

This should be some form of aerobic exercise at least three times a week but preferably five or six. For more details about exercise refer to the paragraphs on spiritual healing in the "Holistic Methods" section of Chapter 4.

Nasalcrom and Cortisone Sprays

At the beginning of this chapter, I mentioned that an awareness of the factors that make sinuses worse is a prerequisite to effectively treating chronic sinusitis. In addition, our indoor air at home is much easier to modify than our outdoor or work environments.

Since most of us spend a considerable amount of time at work and commute there in cars, buses, subways, and trains, we are frequently exposed to harmful factors. Many of us then come home from work and do an aerobic exercise such as running or bicycling, which is not only supposed to help us to become healthier overall but also stimulates the body to produce adrenalin, a natural decongestant. Exercise, therefore, should be a good preventive medicine for chronic sinusitis. But if you're breathing hard and the air you're breathing is visible, I'm not certain that the benefit outweighs the liability. Swimming is another good aerobic exercise. However, chlorine irritates the lining of nasal and sinus membranes — so protect yourself with goggles and nose plugs when swimming in a chlorinated pool.

For the person with chronic sinusitis living in a city and having a daily routine similar to what I've described, having healthier sinuses is a challenge. The saline spray will continue to be a valuable asset if used frequently. But there will be times when the air pollution is so thick you can almost cut it with a knife; when the conference room is filled with cigarette smoke and your clothes smell of it when you come home; when you sit in a traffic jam with the car heater blowing in your face and, opening a window for some "fresh" air, all you're able to breathe is automobile exhaust. These and countless other situations that are similarly harmful to the sinuses call for a stronger dose of preventive medicine.

For several years I recommended any of a number of cortisone nasal sprays, e.g., Nasalide, Beconase, or

Vancenase. More recently I've been using Nasalcrom, which is not cortisone but a topical mast-cell inhibitor. Designed to prevent an allergic reaction from taking place on the nasal mucous membrane, it is not absorbed into the body. It requires several days of use before it's supposed to reach maximum efficacy, but for the purpose described in this chapter it seems to work well following one or two inhalations. Cortisone has both an antiallergic and antiinflammatory effect, and cortisone sprays do have some minimal absorption. These drugs require prescriptions and are used primarily for the treatment of nasal allergies. However, I have substantial empirical evidence from my own experience and that of many of my patients that Nasalcrom or cortisone sprays are quite effective in mitigating the impact of harmful factors affecting sinuses.

One of my good friends, who started as a patient, is Doug Shapiro. He is one of America's top bicycle racers, has been on two U.S. Olympic teams, and is presently riding professionally on the 7-Eleven cycling team. He came to me initially to be treated for a sinus infection. He was concerned that the frequency of these infections was jeopardizing not only his present performance but his future career in cycling. He helped me realize the hazard that cycling, or any other outdoor conditioning sport, poses to the sinuses. There is a tremendous amount of filtering that must be done, because so much more air is presented to the sinuses with the type of breathing that this exercise requires. In addition, there is the drying effect and even the factor of temperature, if it's a cool day. When one is descending a hill at 50 miles an hour on a bicycle, the wind chill factor will produce air that is extremely cold when it hits the mucous membrane.

I began a period of research, essentially using Doug as a guinea pig, to see what we could find that would allow him to ride and remain relatively free of sinus problems. He trained and raced throughout the pollution-choked cities of Europe; in the dryness and altitude of Colorado; in the desert conditions of Baja California. Through cold rain and snow, he routinely rode his bike more than 600 miles a week. We both learned a great deal.

What we found is that the most effective preventive medicine in protecting his sinuses from some of the most demanding conditions that can be imposed on the body's air filter, humidifier, and temperature regulator is Nasalcrom spray. It is most effective when used in anticipation of the harsh conditions, if they can be predicted. Use can take place upon awakening in the morning and again just prior to the exposure. One should first spray with the saline, then blow the nose, then use the Nasalcrom. Remember, this is not something that I'm recommending on a daily basis. It is only to be used when the most harmful conditions for sinuses are present. The cortisone sprays can be used similarly.

Surgery

If you have followed the daily regimen suggested in this chapter for at least three months and are still suffering from repeated sinus infections, then surgery is a possible alternative. You may also be a candidate for surgery if you have been fighting only one acute sinusitis episode over that same period of time. These procedures are performed by Ear, Nose, and Throat (ENT) physicians. This group of doctors are surgeons whose specialty is Otorhinolaryngology.

Sinus surgery may also be performed in those rare instances where an infection spreads beyond the sinus and threatens to cause serious complications. The intraorbital (around and inside the eye socket) and intracranial (in the brain) complications of sinusitis can be serious.

In fact, a recent recommendation made by a Denver pediatrician for any adolescent with frontal sinusitis who has not responded to antibiotic treatment in the first twenty-four hours is that he or she be hospitalized preventively. With the thousands of cases of acute sinusitis I've seen, I've encountered only five instances of intraorbital spread and no instances of intracranial complications. If either of these is present it should be readily apparent. Intraorbital spread can result in swelling of the eyelid, a bulging eyeball, diminished vision, and an inability to move the eye. A person with intracranial complications should exhibit a marked alteration in level of consciousness or ability to think and be alert, along with a very severe headache.

The most common surgical procedures performed on the sinuses are the following: naso-antral windows, Caldwell-Luc operation, and ethmoidectomy. The purpose of these procedures is to allow better drainage and ventilation of the sinuses as well as to remove irreversibly damaged mucosa. The desired objective is for the mucosal lining to return to its normal state. The frequency with which this goal is attained is not high; surgery should not be considered a cure for chronic sinusitis. From my experience with patients who have undergone surgery, they may subsequently experience less discomfort with their sinus infections as a result of better drainage, but often the frequency with which they get the infections is unchanged.

When surgery is performed to eliminate some of the underlying obstructive causes of sinusitis, such as a deviated septum (the partition separating the nostrils), an enlarged or distorted nasal turbinate (ridge), or nasal polyps, then its rate of success is much higher. The occurrence of acute sinusitis following this type of surgery is usually diminished.

CONCLUSION

Treating chronic sinusitis in most parts of the United States will be an ever-increasing challenge. The continued growth of our urban population, with its accompanying plague of air pollution, will be the greatest health risk confronting the majority of Americans and people all over the world in the coming decade. I recently re-read a letter I'd written to Anne Gorsuch in 1981 when she was the head of the Environmental Protection Agency. I described the near-crisis conditions that the air pollution of Denver was creating. Seven years later, in spite of tremendous publicity, a "Better Air Campaign," and the work of several governmental agencies charged with air cleanup, the air in the "Mile-High City" is still filthy, perhaps even worse than before. Automobile emission testing was supposed to make a significant difference, but it hasn't. Diesel cars, the worst of the auto offenders, continue to proliferate without any type of sanction. There has been some minimal progress made on carbon monoxide levels, but the brown cloud is as noxious as ever, and the pollution-alert days continue to be heralded on radio and TV.

Many people in Denver either have a sinus problem themselves or someone in their immediate family does. The National Clean Air Coalition reports that 100 million of us "live in places where the air is so polluted that breathing is hazardous to our health." Our lungs are now in jeopardy, and in addition to an increase in both bronchitis and pneumonia, we are also seeing another disturbing development. Lung cancer has shown the greatest increase of any form of cancer in the United States in the past forty years. This increase is being attributed primarily to cigarettes, but the second most implicated cause is air pollution.

Our sinuses remain the body's chief protector of the lungs. But the sinuses are becoming the weakest part of our bodies, and chronic sinusitis is the most common disease in America. Medical science considers this condition to be incurable. In this chapter I have presented a treatment regimen that I and many of my patients have used for treating our chronic sinus conditions. This program works quite well to both protect and strengthen the weak sinus, to diminish the frequency of acute sinusitis, and to improve quality of life. To summarize, the method is as follows:

— Avoid cigarettes, heavy air pollution, decongestant nasal sprays, and extremely dry and dirty air of any kind.

— Learn the early signs and symptoms of a sinus infection, and treat it quickly if you have one.

— Use humidifiers, saline nasal sprays, and air cleaners on a regular basis.

— Keep Entex and Nasalcrom available and use them as needed, but sparingly.

— Try to eat a healthy diet, take vitamins, and exercise regularly.

— Become more aware of your sinuses and what makes them feel better and worse.

— Whatever practice or technique works for you to enhance your peace of mind and to diminish stress in your life, try to incorporate it into your *daily* life.

If you are interested in going further and believe that it's possible in spite of medical opinions to the contrary, then chronic sinusitis can be cured. I have been able to achieve this for myself by following the recommendations in this chapter, in addition to using the method of spiritual healing described in Chapter 4. With an open mind and the belief that it's possible, you need only to expect it to happen. Remember to have patience and before long you will begin to experience the reality of your affirmation, "My sinuses are now completely healed!"

*For each additional copy,
please send $8.95 (includes shipping)
with your name and address to:
SINUS SURVIVAL
P.O. Box 620236
Littleton, CO 80162-0236*